# Dom's Guide
## To
# Submissive Training
## Vol. 3

How To Use These 31 Everyday Objects To Train Your New Sub For Ultimate Pleasure & Excitement. A Must Read For Any Dom/Master In A BDSM Relationship

Elizabeth Cramer
Copyright© 2013 by Elizabeth Cramer

Copyright© 2013 Elizabeth Cramer
All Rights Reserved.

Warning: The unauthorized reproduction or distribution of this copyrighted work is illegal. No part of this book may be scanned, uploaded or distributed via internet or other means, electronic or print without the author's permission. Criminal copyright infringement without monetary gain is investigated by the FBI and is punishable by up to 5 years in federal prison and a fine of $250,000. (http://www.fbi.gov/ipr/). Please purchase only authorized electronic or print editions and do not participate in or encourage the electronic piracy of copyrighted material.

Publisher: Living Plus Healthy Publishing

ISBN-13: 978-1494487980

ISBN-10: 1494487985

## Disclaimer

The Publisher has strived to be as accurate and complete as possible in the creation of this book. While all attempts have been made to verify information provided in this publication, the Publisher assumes no responsibility for errors, omissions, or contrary interpretation of the subject matter herein. Any perceived slights of specific persons, peoples, or organizations are unintentional.

This book is not intended for use as a source of legal, business, accounting or financial advice. All readers are advised to seek services of competent professionals in the legal, business, accounting, and finance fields.

The information in this book is not intended or implied to be a substitute for professional medical advice, diagnosis or treatment. All content contained in this book is for general information purposes only. Always consult your healthcare provider before carrying on any health program.

# Table of Contents

Introduction ........................................................ 3
Spanking Implements ...................................... 7
   1. Wooden Brushes ........................................ 7
   2. Ping-Pong Paddles & Games Galore .... 10
   3. Rulers ........................................................ 12
   4. Carpet and Rug Beaters............................ 14
   5. Kitchen Utensils ........................................ 16
   6. Window Blind Rods ................................ 18
   7. Good Ol' Fashioned Switch .................... 20
   8. Build a Chamois Flogger.......................... 22
   9. Build a Hard Rubber Flogger ................ 24
Training and Fun.............................................. 27
   10. Pen and Paper ........................................ 27
   11. Body Marking ........................................ 30
   12. Floor or Car Mats.................................... 32
   13. Kneel On Rice ........................................ 34
   14. Chopsticks and Rubber Bands............ 36

15. Alternative Clamp Resources ............... 38
16. Analgesic Cream ..................................... 40
17. Candle Wax ............................................. 42
18. Ginger ...................................................... 44
19. Collar and Leash .................................... 46
20. Chastity Envelopes ................................ 48
21. Plumber's Twine .................................... 50
    Bondage Necessities ................................ 53

22. Rope ......................................................... 53
23. A Jump Rope ........................................... 55
24. Cling Wrap .............................................. 56
25. Scarves ..................................................... 58
26. Panties ..................................................... 59
27. The Belt ................................................... 61
28. Boxing Gloves ......................................... 63
29. Sleeping Bag ........................................... 65
30. Pool Noodles ........................................... 66
31. Your Sofa ................................................. 67
Conclusion ....................................................... 69

# Introduction

Any visit to a BDSM fetish site, Reddit subgroup or D/s Tumblr will convince you that every Master has a huge house filled with either gothic décor or fluffy white couches, and a ridiculously full selection of paddles, straps, whips, crops, restraints, sex toys, and bondage gear.

Most of those photos come from one of the many franchises owned by Kink.com, the largest US producer of fetish videos and photography, and they really do have a warehouse filled with every leather strap and fancy contraption imaginable. But, what about the average local Doms? Most of them have a special paddle or two, their big, heavy hands, and the belt which holds their pants up. There has to be something better.

Fortunately, you don't have to pay a hundred dollars for a specialty flogger or purchase a wedge from Extreme Restraints for three hundred bucks in order to be a great Dom and provide your sub with hours of bondage, spanking and fun. Most of the things you need to give your submissive the spanking of a lifetime, a punishment to fit the crime, or just an incredible bondage experience can be found right in your own home. Your sub will not only enjoy the variety of experiences in her sessions but also appreciate your creativity.

Aside from the cost savings, there is another benefit to using everyday objects in your BDSM training and session fun – discretion. Not every person can be seen walking down the street or through an airport with a leather whip in his hand or a wooden paddle in his bag. Many Doms must conceal their activities from employers, social circles, or vanilla spouses. Common objects make it easier to engage in important rituals without detection.

Asking your sub to keep a wooden hairbrush in her purse won't bring up anything suspicious and you can take quite a few rulers, Ping-Pong paddles or scarves on your trip without the TSA raising a red flag.

This guide is designed to give you 31 common objects you already own or can purchase for minimal cost and keep right out in the open that will enhance your BDSM relationship and provide you and your sub hours of pleasure.

There are three categories represented in the guide: **spanking implements**, **training and fun items**, and **bondage necessities**.

Let's get started!

# Spanking Implements

### 1. Wooden Brushes

Let's face it – even the heaviest, most experienced hand starts to hurt eventually. If you have a sub with a high pain tolerance it is likely her bottom could outlast the sensitive skin on your palm.

All spanking implements specialize in one of two sensations – thud or sting. Implements that "thud" tend to be heavier and create a deep impact, often leaving bruising. "Stinging" implements are more flexible and weigh less. Their impact is mostly felt on top of the skin and they create a stinging/burning sensation that is more immediately painful than a thud but does very little lasting damage.

The hand is a thudding implement. In order to provide a well-rounded spanking, a stinging implement should also be used so your sub can experience the immediate sting of the spanking for the first few hours, but also feel the bruising throughout the day.

Wooden hairbrushes are made of light quality wood (women don't want to carry around a one pound hairbrush) so the flat back surface of the brush provides an excellent form of sting.

Hairbrushes are also naturally made to fit the hand well, and some even include a sort-of shock absorbing neck design that keeps the hand from feeling the full force of the recoiling vibration. Best of all, no one ever accused someone of being kinky because they had a hairbrush in their desk drawer (although, if you are bald – you might want to ask her to hang on to it).

For self-spanking (if you aren't able to be with your sub all the time and want to ensure she is able to get a few good licks every morning) or for a swatting experience closer to that of a large paddle, try a long handled wooden bath brush. Bath brushes are designed for people to be able to reach those "unreachable" places when washing, and they do just as well for spanking.

The long handle also lets the Dom take a position farther from the sub's bottom which gives him a chance for a full arm swing. Bath brushes have a little more thud than a hairbrush, but do provide a nice point of impact.

## 2. Ping-Pong Paddles & Games Galore

Vanilla people never seem to notice this, but the world is full of natural paddles. Even the games we play come with a variety of tools which can be co-opted into spanking implements without complication.

The most obvious paddle is, of course, the Ping-Pong paddle. These little round paddles come with so many choices there are a variety of sensations that can be produced with little or no alteration. The standard Ping-Pong paddle has a small handle and a round surface covered by a thin, bumpy rubber material. It provides a balance between sting and thud.

If you pull the protective rubber sheet off of each side, you get a solid wood paddle that has a great thud. Many Doms choose to remover the rubber from one side and leave it on the other to get two different responses from the same implement. They also make Ping-Pong paddles with thicker rubber on the surface (more sting), or made entirely of hard plastic (ultimate sting!).

If you don't have any reason to have a Ping-Pong paddle around, or desire even more choices – go to the table tennis or racquet sports aisle of any sporting goods store. There are novelty game paddles, wall-ball paddles, and even paddles made out of nerf material (those don't sting or thud, but they are fun to play with).

Beyond the sporting goods section, you can always head over to the toy department (particularly around Easter) and pick up a classic child's paddle ball toy. This is a light wooden paddle (sting) with a rubber band and a ball attached to it. Pull off the band/ball combo and you have a perfect, hand sized, light wooden paddle.

Because it is a child's toy the wood can be flimsy so small light strokes are going to work better than big heavy whacks which will crack the paddle in half. Then again, breaking a paddle on your sub's behind might just add a little spark to your evening.

## 3. Rulers

While you're walking around the store putting together a vast menagerie of spanking implements, don't forget to stop by the school/office department and pick up the teacher's old standby – the ruler.

Don't bother with the thin, plastic rulers on sale for fifty cents. Even the clear solid ones will break in the first two minutes. Instead, chose one of the flexible metal rulers. If you can't find those on the school supply aisle go over to where office supplies are kept or stop by an office supply store.

Metal rulers have a number of advantages. They don't break, even with repeated hard snaps, and they come in different lengths from 6 to 18 inches. The best part is their flexible nature. If you have an 18 inch ruler you can smack your sub's rear and "sit spot" (that area of flesh at the very bottom of the buttocks that makes contact with the chair when she sits down) and the end of the ruler will wrap around her body and provide a sharp sting to her hips or the side of her cheeks as well.

Wooden rulers do not make good spanking implements on the bottom due to the extreme light weight of the wood (many are made of reinforced balsa wood), but can be used to smack the inside of the open hand.

If you have a sub who is prone to using her middle finger as a communication tool – a few swift smacks on the palm with a wooden ruler will change that habit in a hurry.

## 4. Carpet and Rug Beaters

For a lovely sting that will not only redden your sub's bottom in record time but also leave a delightful pattern of swirls and arcs on her as well, there's nothing better than a carpet beater (also known as a rug beater).

These light rods are usually made out of rattan, a material similar to the bamboo of a cane. They have a long handle then blossom out into a clover-shaped head with space and swirls. Heavy enough to beat the dust off a living room rug, when used at handle-length and given a good swat, carpet beaters can bruise heavily and create a lot of thud.

If you stand closer to your sub (draping her over a sofa arm or chair) and use it lightly making rapid strokes back and forth, it will be more of a stinging implement and provide her with some hot cheeks very quickly.

Carpet beaters, particularly antique ones, are pretty enough that some folks hang them in the kitchen or spare room as part of the décor. Imagine how much fun it would be to entertain your boss for dinner, knowing the tool you use to spank your submissive is hanging on the wall behind him.

There are modern carpet beaters made out of coiled wire on the market as well. Those should be avoided for punishment as the metal has no flexibility and could cut or injure your sub.

## 5. Kitchen Utensils

Once you become a Dom, you'll never walk through the kitchen utensil aisle of a store and look at those items the same way again. Modern kitchens contain a cornucopia of spanking implements.

The first that generally comes to mind is the one many a mom reached for when she discovered a transgression while cooking dinner – the spatula. Made of a hard plastic, usually with some holes to allow air flow, with a perfect length handle, spatulas are a natural spanking implement. Depending on the flexibility of the plastic they can provide sting or thud.

The other kitchen implement already famous as a spanking item of choice is the wooden spoon. Made of balsa wood, or sometimes heartier stuff, wooden spoons can redden a bottom and give a boiling red sting in no time. They require a lot of arm effort due to the lightness, but definitely raise the hue of your sub to a solid red quickly and persuasively.

Beyond the two obvious choices, the kitchen aisle is a veritable playground of options. Cake icers are long thin tools with a one inch wide flexible metal sheath on them. They make fantastic spanking tools (similar to a metal ruler) and can be used on the hands or breasts as well.

Other than spanking, salad tongs can be used for breast torture, stirring spoons with the wide angle head made great pussy spankers, and with a lot of lube – a turkey baster can add some fun as well. If you're looking for an evening with a little imagination – take yourself to the cooking store.

## 6. Window Blind Rods

Besides maintenance spanking and erotic fun, every sub needs correction now and then. Nothing helps your sub learn better or respond quicker than a good judicial caning. Whether you prefer the British correctional protocol (6 of the best!) or the Asian judicial method a few strokes with a cane will leave a definite impression on your sub.

Because caning is not popular in the US, it can be costly and inconvenient to acquire a punishment cane. It's not the kind of thing most Doms want showing up in the mail. Do not attempt to discipline your submissive with an American walking cane. The wood is too sturdy and thick (they are made to hold a person's weight) and will injure your sub.

One suitable replacement for the effect of the cane can be found hanging from your window seal. Most window blinds, including mini blinds, come with a plastic rod that hangs down from the blind used to open and close the slats. They are often attached with a simple plastic hook and can be removed and replaced easily.

The rod is the right length and substance to give your sub a few good strokes. Unlike thinner wooden dowels, the rod will not break or leave splinters in your sub's rear end. Being made of plastic also means the rod will provide a high amount of sting.

As a good Dom you always want to adhere to the oath you took with your submissive – you will "hurt but not harm" her. As such, start very lightly with the rod until you get a good feel for how much pain it can deliver and the best way to handle it.

Give your sub a quick warm-up hand spanking first to give her a little help in adjusting to the sharp pain, then hold the rod no more than 3 to 6 inches from her bottom and give her a few good snaps. If she doesn't feel that it is painful enough, try holding it out a little farther and keep trying until you get the best length and power angle for her punishment.

Trust me, soon the term "Window Treatment" will have a whole new meaning in your house.

## 7. Good Ol' Fashioned Switch

For sheer punishment American style nothing beats the good old-fashioned switch. There are a lot of plusses to switches. If you live in a wooded area – they are free (they literally grow on trees) and they provide a cutting sting that can reduce the most stubborn pain resistant sub to tears. Switches also have a natural built-in ritual quality to them that makes them a very powerful ally in training your sub.

The longest walk in the world is the walk your sub will make, in silence, to pick her own switch and bring it back to you. It's one thing to be punished. It's another level of anticipation when you realize you are choosing the rod that will be used on you.

Have your sub leave any leaves, twigs or off-shoots on the switch. Stand in front of her while you peel off the attachments so she can watch you prepare the switch and transform it from a stick to a punishment rod. This is also a good time to engage in any lecturing you want to do. By the time she is bent over and ready for her punishment, she will already be shaking with anticipation and fear.

The best use for a switch isn't on the behind (although it can do a lot of stinging there), but the back of the legs and calves. Make sure to grab your sub by the arm or hold her torso if she's over your lap so she can't kick or pull away from the vicious sting.

If you don't live in an area with trees, take your sub on a picnic or a "switch hunting" trip where you can visit somewhere that does offer trees you can use to collect a few good switches for home. Keep those switches on top of the fridge (unless company is coming over) or dresser and have her retrieve one when it's time for correction.

When at all possible, a fresh flexible switch cut directly from a tree is better than a dry switch. Fresh switches give more sting and are less likely to break.

## 8. Build a Chamois Flogger

Spanking isn't just about learning or punishment, there's also an erotic component to it as well. When it's not time for the punishment or maintenance spanking, a sultry erotic flogging is in order.

Floggers come in two main categories – soft and hard. Soft floggers generally have at least 3 or more "tails" made of a loose or pliant material that provides a gentle sting on the skin. With repeated strokes heat can build up on the body, but it is clearly more of a sensual experience.

Hard floggers are made of stiff leather, rubber, or light wood like rattan and can have one "tail" or many. Hard floggers have more thud than sting and can sometimes be a cutting tool as well. Hard floggers are still designed to provide sexual pleasure, but are used more for masochists with a high pain tolerance and edge play.

To make a soft flogger, go somewhere that sells supplies for washing cars and buy a large soft chamois. Cut the chamois into long thin strips, about 1/4 of an inch wide. You can leave a few strips as wide as a half inch if you want to have variety in the touch points of the flogger.

Head on over to the bicycle aisle and purchase a pair of bicycle handlebar grips (you'll need one for this flogger, and one for the next on the list). The hard rubber grips work a lot better than the foam ones.

Group together your strips of chamois and string them through the hole in the bottom of the handlebar grip. Split them into two sections and tie a knot to keep them attached to the grip. You can also use a little superglue to hold the knot in place or firm up the hole in the grip.

The result is a nice soft flogger that cost much less than you would pay at a fetish store, and shows your sub you're willing to put effort into things to delight her.

## 9. Build a Hard Rubber Flogger

When you are on the bicycle aisle getting handlebar grips, pick up a couple of bicycle inner-tubes while you are at it. The inner tube is the small cheap tube that goes inside the larger tire. They come in small boxes and cost around three dollars. The rubber is thin enough to cut with a good pair of household scissors.

Cut the lining of one or two inner tubes (depending on the number of tails you want) into 1/4 inch strips (no larger) and gather them together. Pull them through the handlebar grip until the ends go through the small hole at the end of the grip and separate them into two sections. Tie the sections together in a knot. You can use superglue or a lighter to melt the ends together (similar to patching a bike tire) to form a solid anchor.

The rubber flogger is going to have a lot more sting than the soft flogger and can damage your sub's skin if it hits with too much force. Start with soft strokes without too much snap and raise the intensity slowly until you get a feel for what kind of pain she can tolerate.

If you want to add more bite – take the time to take 3 of the strips and braid them together to form a tail similar to a single tail whip. If you have 9 strips you can make a 3 tail whip that will increase the thud and potential for cutting into the skin.

# Training and Fun

Successfully training your sub will require more than just spanking and corporal punishment. There are a number of creative ways you two can play, learn and develop as a BDSM couple using common items and creative energy.

## 10. Pen and Paper

One of the undeniable truths about BDSM is that it's almost impossible to punish a masochist. The more you heap on her, the more she loves it. So, traditional spanking becomes more of a reward than a correction tool. For women like that, or just to add variety to your training regimen, a classic punishment will do the trick. In a Master's hands, pen and paper can be a tool bringing absolute remorse.

Writing lines isn't a new idea. School teachers used it for a hundred years to teach students how to behave in the classroom and encourage good penmanship at the same time. Like corner time, the power of writing lines is found in how utterly boring and pointless it is.

In the late 1980's in the US, English teachers decided it was wrong to punish students by making them write (something they were trying to encourage students to enjoy) and the practice fell out of favor. However, it is perfectly suited to correct any willing slave, activity junkie, or Daddy's little sub.

For correction, give your sub a good hard spanking (or at least redden her bottom a bit) and sit her on a hard wooden chair (or punishment mat – to be discussed later) with paper and pen in front of her. Assign her a line to write 100, 500, or a consequential amount of times (for example: if she gets a ticket that costs 85.00 have her write 85 lines - or 850). The line should be long, with labor intensive words and illustrative of the punishment.

Ex: I will not ignore my Master's instructions and go over the speed limit on Interstate 64.

Require her to use perfect penmanship or printing. Use a red marker to circle any word that goes off the line, any period or capitalization missed and assign one swat per error.

If you are a Daddy Dom working with a Little Girl you might want to get the "learning my letters" notepads for children and a large pencil to write her lines, or make her write with her non-dominant hand (left handed for right handers, etc.).

## 11. Body Marking

The human body is more than the vehicle our souls wander around inside. It is the physical manifestation of our identity. Your submissive has spent her lifetime thinking of her breasts, her ass, her arms and legs as the very incarnation of who she is as a woman. How better to transform her thinking during training than to mark that property as your own?

Any common marker or highlighter can be used for body marking or writing. You can write your name across her breasts or put an invitation for use on her butt cheeks. With her consent, a play and picture session can be both educational and erotic.

Do not use a Sharpie on your sub if she has to go to work or has a vanilla/unaware spouse at home. A Sharpie soaks into the pores and takes a few days and a lot of scrubbing to get completely out.

For quick use that is easy to get off the skin, try dry erase markers. The marks don't come off as easily as they do on a dry erase board, but a little soap and water will wash all the evidence away.

A variation of body marking for more sexual purposes is to use syrup to write upon your lover's skin. Maple syrup is a lot of fun to write with because it will leave your sub good and sticky as well.

If you write clearly, and want to use this as a punishment, you can write on her with maple syrup then cover it with flour. The flour will dry on the syrup creating a sticky/clear impression, but it's all washed away with a dip in the bathtub.

Use chocolate syrup for words you plan to "lick off" her skin or dip a clean/washed paintbrush in the syrup and put your own edible mark upon her.

## 12. Floor or Car Mats

Punishments don't have to be fast or active to provide an intense lesson. In fact, this punishment works wonders if you are an online Dom or have to spend time away from your submissive. She can obediently punish herself creating almost as much pain as you do with a little time.

The next time you are in an office, or office supply store, look at the plastic mats used under chairs to protect the carpet. On the top, they are smooth plastic so the chair can run over them easily. On the bottom they have a host of plastic nubs or spikes designed the keep the mat in place by digging into the carpet. Car floor mats have the same properties. Now, imagine those nubs digging into the bare bottom of your sub over time. It definitely makes an impression.

Cut an office mat into the size and shape of the chair or stool your sub will be sitting on. Give her an amount of time she is to sit naked from the waist down on the mat. To begin with, 15 or 30 minutes is a good start. You can combine the pain of the mat with writing an essay or writing lines, if this is a specific punishment.

Once your sub sits on the mat the immediate pain will seem to go away after a few minutes. Then she will feel intermittent pulses and soreness beginning to develop. The maximum pain will happen when you release her from the mat. The nubs dig into the skin and she will have to "peel" the mat off of her, leaving indentures where the nubs were.

The act of removing the mat is nearly as painful as the moment the sub sits down. If you have assigned this as a self-punishment, have your sub send you a picture of her bottom after rising from the mat so the red marks will prove her obedience.

If you want to make the punishment harsher, seat your sub on a chair that is so high her feet do not touch the floor. This will put extra pressure on her bottom on the mat. You can also increase the pressure by adding a harder surface, like a block of wood, or stack of books underneath the mat to lift it into her body.

Finally, if you really want to challenge your sub, have her sit down and stand up off the mat (the two most painful moments) at 10 minute intervals, until she begs you to stop or a set number of repetitions has occurred.

## 13. Kneel On Rice

If having a mat is not practical or your sub gets accustomed to that process, there is another sure way to use time to get her attention. Require your sub to kneel on uncooked rice. Like the nubs on the mat, the rice digs into the very tender skin on the knees and calves causing a sharp initial pain and ache afterward. Many women claim they have had enough after five minutes on the rice, and will beg to be let up quickly.

Kneeling on rice is a great punishment for training a kitchen sub or correcting a sub who is derelict in her duties in domestic service. It also has a nice ritual component to it.

Measure out a cup or two of rice and pour it with a good concentration of rice in a small square (12 inches by 12 inches is good) on the floor. If you want, you can use masking tape to make the square and leave it on the floor for a while before the punishment so every time she sees the square she knows what is coming.

Have your sub stand in front of the square and recite the reasons for her punishment, or a litany of devotion to you. At your finger snap or command have her kneel on the rice.

Set a kitchen timer behind her back where she cannot see how much time you put on it, and place it near her. That way she will be hoping it will ding, signifying the end of her time. Teach her not to stand when the timer goes off, but to ask your permission to stand. When she does she can brush the rice off of her legs with her hands.

If you want to challenge your sub, give her a pair of chopsticks and have her pick up the rice and put it in a bowl then carry it to the trash and throw it away. Assign one swat for every grain she misses.

## 14. Chopsticks and Rubber Bands

Picking up rice isn't the only punishment in which chopsticks are put to good use. With their linear construction and thin exterior, chopsticks make the perfect tool for providing varying levels of pressure. You can use chopsticks and rubber bands to clamp around most body parts and put either small or painful pressure on sensitive areas.

To use chopsticks on breasts, have your sub kneel (on rice or not) before you while you kiss, lightly bite or arouse her so her nipples stand erect then place one chopstick underneath her nipple and the other on top. Use the rubber bands to hold the sticks together.

You can determine the pressure/pain on the nipples in two ways. You can loosen the rubber bands which will lower the pressure on the nipple. You can also determine the level of pain based on where you put the chopsticks. If you put them lower toward the breasts where you include most of the nipple and areola, the pain will be less. If you put the chopsticks more forward on the breast to where they are simply pinching the tip of the nipple, the pain will be much more extensive.

One of the nice things about using this and other alternative clamps is the extra humiliation the sub experiences at the punishment. Kneeling in expensive silver nipple clamps will make your sub feel trained and garnished, like a pony girl. Kneeling in a pair of chopsticks (particularly if you get the free bamboo ones you can pick up at any Chinese food take-out place) held together by rubber bands is embarrassing and ups the emotion of the punishment.

## 15. Alternative Clamp Resources

While chopsticks and rubber bands certainly are a visual and painful experience for your sub, your house is full of all kinds of plentiful, natural clamping devices that can be put to use for training, sex and fun.

The most obvious clamp is the clothespin. Like the chopsticks mentioned before, the further into the breast you clip a clothespin the lighter the pain will be. The nice thing about clothespins is that you get about 40 or 50 in one bag.

You can place the clips in a circle around your sub's areola (this is great if she happens to have particularly large areolas). After leaving her for a set amount of time for the pain to set in, ask her to recite a litany, oath or promise she made to you for each clip. Take them off one by one. Alternately, you can slap the clips off, which gives the sensitive tissue a quick pinch before falling off your sub.

Potato chip bag closers are a close cousin to the clothespin. These plastic clamps are also more versatile and have a larger range than the average clothespin. You can use two chip bag closers to help in training your sub to keep her legs open for you. Position her legs in an open position and place one clip on each side of her labia. Set a certain number of minutes on the timer and have her speak a litany about the sub's promise to be always open to the Master.

Finally, if you are fond of nipple clamps that hook together on a chain and pull the breasts toward one another in such a way that slapping one breast pulls on the other, there is a solution for that as well.

Go to your sub's closet (or a store) and get a skirt hanger. Skirt hangers are regular hangers with two clamps on the bottom bar so a skirt can hang evenly from them. Most skirt hangers have adjustable clamps so you can slide them in order to get the right length. Slide the clamps into a position that allows you to clip both breasts with one hanger.

## 16. Analgesic Cream

One of the challenges of being a 24/7 Master is finding ways for your sub to fill the downtime so you don't have to be constantly stimulating or working with her. The challenge for an online Dom is finding ways for your sub to be punished or stimulated while you are far away. One quick answer to both of those problems can be found in your medicine cabinet or in any drugstore: analgesic cream.

Analgesic cream, often sold under such names as Icy Hot, BenGay, or Mineral Ice, was created for the purpose of loosening up stiff muscles and reducing pain by providing the sensation of warmth or cold on the skin. The creams don't actually change the skin temperature at all, but the chemicals in the cream provide the sensation of change which travels up the nerves and overrides the pain impulse in the brain.

Creams that provide a cold sensation use menthol; the ones used to provide a burning/heat sensation use capsaicin (the same ingredient found in chili peppers). When applied to more sensitive parts of the body, analgesic creams can give your sub a sexy or punishing sensation requiring little action on your part. Used in combination with spanking or other training methods, it can create additional stimuli for your sub to endure.

Require your sub to rub the cream on her nipples or rim of her outer labia (NEVER the inner labia). If you are an online Dom, have her do this while instant messaging you then describe the feelings online as the sensation grows. If it gets too hot (or too cold) for her to handle, she can beg for you to allow her to wash it off.

If you are punishing your sub in person, give her a hard reddening spanking, then rub the cream on her bottom and send her to corner time with the instruction not to touch or rub herself. You will get to see a good version of the "spanking dance" as the sensations overtake her behind.

Make sure to wash your hands after handling the cream. Follow directions with regard to the number of applications and amount of time between applications provided by the manufacturer.

## 17. Candle Wax

It is hot and punishing, tests the bonds of trust and pain tolerance, and an act of pure submission to receive – yet nothing is more visually erotic than dripping hot wax onto your sub. Depending on your relationship and sense of arousal, you can restrain her to a bed and blindfold her so she isn't sure when each drop is going to land, or have her kneel before you and ask you for each drop, knowing what is coming. There are important things to know about dripping hot wax on a partner.

The best wax to use is paraffin wax. It has a lower melting point and will not be as hot or dangerous to the skin as regular candle wax. Use "soft candles" such as a paraffin pillar or candles with mineral oil inside – like the kind that come in glass jars – for dripping. Do not use dinner table tapers, beeswax or emergency candles which have a much higher boiling point. They can injure your partner.

If you are just beginning with wax play, place a piece of plastic wrap (such as saran wrap) over your partner so she can get used to the heat without incurring any risk.

Make sure to put a plastic sheet or old towel/sheet under your partner before playing with wax. Light the candle and let each drop fall on her. You can also collect several drops on a spoon and ladle them on her, letting the stream drip down. If you find candles of different colors you can turn your beloved into a work of art.

To remove the wax, you can let it dry and remove it with a fingernail file, dull edge instrument (like a putty knife or spatula) or just pick it off. If your sub has trouble removing it, there is solvent sold in the same kits as wax hair removal products that will help dissolve the wax. After it is off, a quick shower is all that's needed.

## 18. Ginger

There are a number of ways to play with your food and have good sex at the same time. However, one root is not only sexy and tasty – it was made to stimulate and train your partner.

Using peeled ginger root (sometimes called "figging" or "ginger figging") in your partner's vagina or anus will cause an itching/burning sensation that increases lubrication, desire and pleasure/pain.

In "Pony Play" a small dab of ginger jelly or slice of ginger is sometimes added to the "tail" (butt plug) to make the pony step livelier or show more enthusiasm.

Ginger figging has an interesting history. It was originally used in Victorian England as a court appointed punishment for "wayward women." The burn comes from the essential oil in the ginger root and is harmless in the long-term. But, when your sub's bottom is stinging and rocking from it, don't ask her if it feels harmless!

On a traditional pain scale the pain is about a 1 or 2, but the itching and desire for movement to relieve it is about a 4. The fresher the ginger root, the more sting/pain occurs.

Go to the produce section and buy a piece of ginger root. The way the "fingers" are shaped, it already looks like a sexual device. When you are ready to play, use a paring knife and peel the brown skin off the root, revealing the flesh of the ginger.

If you are going to insert the root as a butt plug, make sure you carve it with a recessed base (like a traditional butt plug) so that it doesn't get sucked into the anal cavity and require a trip to the doctor to remove.

Insert the root with a little lube into her anus. The burn will begin to manifest. Encourage her to try to last through the first few minutes as the pain will subside into an ember. If she can't, remove the root. She'll still feel the sensation for a while.

You can also cut the root into small wedges to insert vaginally or near her clitoris (for a few seconds only). Make sure after peeling the root you wash your hands thoroughly because you will have the oil on your hands and you don't want to accidently rub your eyes or mouth.

Experiment with areas, time durations, and activities (spanking while a root is inserted) until you find the right balance of pleasure and pain for your sub.

## 19. Collar and Leash

It goes without saying that a sub should be collared in a temporary collar the moment she offers her submission to you. However, if you go online you'll notice those fancy leather "slave" collars can be quite costly and take several weeks to be mailed to your home.

Usually, if a commitment comes quickly, you don't want to wait three weeks to collar your sub. There are also occasions for training or punishment when you don't want her in a fancy collar, but want to objectify or remove her status for training or punishment. There are many alternatives to a slave collar from a fetish site.

Most people find training collars, either leather or nylon, at the pet store. Prices vary from the expensive fancy leather collars, to the cheaper nylon/plastic clip collars. If you are engaging in puppy play or simply want a low-end training collar for your sub's workout – a nylon collar will work very well. You can even drop a buck or two in the tag machine by the door of most pet shops and have a custom-made tag for your sub's collar.

If you don't like the pet shop look, use a piece of ribbon. There are many colors to choose from and you can use the colors to show meanings, match your slave's nail polish or go with the season. You can buy a small spool of ribbon at any general store. Cut a long enough piece of ribbon to fit snugly around your sub's neck and leave enough of a tail to tie a bow. If you or your sub can tie pretty bows – leave the bow up front. If not, tie it into a knot and leave it under her hair in the back.

For a quick collar and leash – you can always use tie downs (like a kayak tie down rope or a mover's tie down). Make sure the clip of the tie down is firm because you don't want it to slide down and choke your sub. Anytime your sub advises you the collar is pulling too tightly or restricting her breathing, you must loosen it. The same trick with pets (at least 2 fingers fit under the collar) works for subs as well.

## 20. Chastity Envelopes

One of the first things you will train your sub is that her sexuality is your property and she is not to engage in self-satisfying behaviors without your expressed permission.

Taking control of your submissive's sexual expression is one of the foundations of a power exchange relationship. As such, one of the most powerful tools you have at your disposal is enforced chastity.

Chastity training gets to the core of who you are as the Master and how much she can endure to honor your wishes. It is also a good way to build both trust and anticipation.

There are a number of ways to have fun and engage in enforced chastity (or orgasm denial) in your relationship that don't involve a steel belt locked around her waist. Use sealed envelopes to create a little mystery and anticipation in your sub.

Get a decorative bowl, or pretty box, as a gift for your sub. Cut 30 pieces of paper into small squares. On five of the papers write the word "YES!" On five more papers write the word "ASK!" (that means it could be a yes or a no, depending on your response to her asking), and on 20 of the papers write "Not Today." Fold and mix them all up. Each day you see her, allow your sub to reach into her box and pull out a paper. In training, you can also have her do something to earn a chance to reach into the box or as a punishment take a chance away to reach into the box. Remind her she has a 1 in 3 chance of getting a positive response.

The other thing you can do is write down the number of days until she has your permission to reach a climax or touch herself (if you are an online Dom). Include a poem or treat of some kind. Seal that number in a thick envelope and leave it with her. Give her a chance each day to guess the number. If she guesses right, she can have your permission that day. If she guesses wrong, she has to wait until the actual number of days pass. Then, allow her to open the envelope on the assigned day.

## 21. Plumber's Twine

Although the last time they were popular was the 12th century, chastity belts for women have been making a surprising resurgence in the last ten years thanks to the internet and rise in BDSM community culture. There are countless websites devoted to women who wear chastity belts or couples who use chastity as part of their D/s experience.

The belts themselves have improved over the centuries and are now made of stainless steel with a screen to allow the wearer to comfortably use the bathroom and in-seam locks to make them less bulky. Still, for all the advances chastity belts have a lot of issues.

They are expensive. A generic belt can cost between $400 - $600 dollars and a fitted one with in-seam locks is closer to $1,500 and can take 6 months to arrive. There are cheap knock-offs for about $80.00 but they fall apart at the first wearing and are really more of a costume than the real thing.

Modern chastity belts are also sized for smaller women with 10 or 12 being the largest measurement possible, and no matter how smoothly the lock sets in, they are still bulky and impossible to wear underneath clothing without being detected.

Fortunately there is a way to remind your sub of her chastity, give her a little arousal to keep her on edge, fits any size and it won't cost more than five dollars.

Plumber's twine is thick brown twine used by plumbers to create a plumb line. It is wiry but flexible and easy to work with. Have your sub (or better yet – do this yourself) wrap the twine around her waist, right above the hips and cut enough twine so she has two ends with which to tie a knot so it makes a sort of belt around her waist.

Then take a second piece of twine and tie it to the belt in the front, guide it through her labia and pull it snug – so the twine rubs up against the clitoral hood. Bring it between her legs and tie it to the back of the belt (making sure to pull the string tight).

The twine offers a constant reminder of her chastity, but she can use the bathroom, wear it under her clothing, and it will rub her clitoral hood all day keeping her in a state of near arousal. When her time of chastity is over – just cut the string.

# Bondage Necessities

### 22. Rope

Whether you are into bondage or rope play, every Dom needs a length of good hearty rope around. Different types of rope exists for different things and it can be purchased cheaply in just about any store.

The best rope for bondage is soft nylon rope. Not only is it woven to be particularly strong, but the softness of the actual fiber keeps from cutting into your sub's skin.

Besides the inexpensive cost, rope has the advantages of being versatile enough that you can cut it or shape it for any length and it has a myriad of uses. You can use rope to tie your sub to a bed or keep her in a preferred position. You can also engage in strict rope play and spend hours knotting and positioning her as decoratively as possible.

Rope can create a make-shift collar and lead (just make sure knots you tie are solid and do not slip or choke your sub) or can be used to hold a gag in place, or wrapped between her legs to hold a dildo or plug in the right spot.

Whether you're tying, spanking, holding, or guiding – a little bit of rope can go a long, long way.

## 23. A Jump Rope

A rope by any other name – is still a rope. Jump ropes are steadily climbing in popular use as adults have discovered the popular children's toy can bring as much health and fitness to them in adulthood as it did during their youth. Besides strengthening the legs and heart, jump ropes can make the BDSM heart grow fonder.

Jump ropes can be used to train and restrain a sub, and unlike other restraining objects include a ball of regular rope – jump ropes look perfectly normal in a suitcase or gym bag. A lot of adults travel with jump ropes as a form of portable fitness so the airport security personnel won't blink twice when they see a jump rope go by. Of course, once you're at your destination, you can use the rope to tie your sub's hands or feet and no one will be the wiser.

Beyond the nylon rope, you can also get the plastic type children use. When doubled in your hand, a plastic jump rope makes a great whipping tool and provides a lot of sting. Jump ropes are also great for games or competitions between subs and make a nice toy for the room if you engage in Daddy/Little one play.

## 24. Cling Wrap

An essential for most kitchens, cling wrap, sold under such names as Saran Wrap or Clear Plastic Wrap, is also a must for every Dom's play room. You can use cling wrap to cover your sub's skin (so you can still see her) in order to protect her during wax play, paint play, etc.

Cling wrap is light enough to be used as a protective covering for cuts or wounds until your play period is over (when the wound needs to be washed and bandaged properly) and strong enough to be used for bondage.

If you wrap cling wrap around your sub's wrists with enough revolutions it is impossible to pull apart. Make sure to keep sharp scissors around for any session where you intend to use cling wrap to secure a sub or restrain her to an object. You will not be able to unwrap her without help.

The other attraction to cling wrap in BDSM is mummification. With enough wrap you can immobilize your partner and wrap her up tight. Make sure you are not wrapping over her mouth, or wrapping so tightly you are constricting her ability to breathe by compressing her lungs.

Cling wrap will stick to her naked body due to the natural oils in her skin, and you'll still be able to see her and admire your sub.

## 25. Scarves

Versatile, sexy and strong – scarves are a perfect tool for D/s games and sessions with your sub. If you meet your sub in her office after hours or want to have a quickie in the back of your SUV, you can still add some excitement by using the scarf she wore for the day.

Scarves can be used as blindfolds to place over her eyes and take her on a trust walk or just give her the chance to focus solely on pleasing you by limiting her vision and distractions. A wide or layered scarf is best for a blindfold so it covers enough of her face to keep her from peeking through the bottom.

Scarves can also be used to secure a soft gag in the mouth of your sub, or as a light gag to wrap around her mouth. Put a scarf in her mouth then hold her head by holding both ends of the scarf while using her from behind. They make great impromptu tie down devices with a softer touch.

If you are meeting a new sub who is hesitant about cuffs or leather, a scarf is a fantastic start. Best of all, scarves are something that can be worn in public, taken on airplanes and don't invite judgment on you or your sex life.

## 26. Panties

During training and into submission, your sub's panties are usually one of the first things to come off. Before you discard the silky covering as an unwanted device, take a moment to think of all the things you can do with your partner's panties.

Ask any submissive woman and she will tell you she prefers a soft gag over all the others (ball gag, penis gag, leather bit) and the sexiest gag of all is to have her Master pull off her panties and stuff them in her mouth. The act is demeaning, alluring, personal and undeniably dominant. Secure the panties with her scarf and you have a great gag.

During a spanking ritual, it is effective to spank a submissive over her panties to give her a warm up, then peel them down to bare her bottom. The act stimulates the feelings of power exchange. To add to the humiliation, leave her panties around her knees or ankles. That provides the "little girl" feeling of shame she's been looking for and also restrains how far her legs can kick or move.

If your submissive is new and in training, her panties can easily be used as a reward (particularly if she is uncomfortable being naked so much of the time). Explain to your sub that panties are a privilege, and she must earn the right to be covered in your site or sleep in them. In the hands of an experienced Dom, panties are an amazing tool.

## 27. The Belt

To a submissive woman there is no sound more seductive than the hiss of a leather belt pulling through your pant loops and being doubled in your hand. In fact, some women endure a belt spanking just to experience the chills of that moment of sweet anticipation. Utilize your belt to its full potential by building to that moment and accentuating it as much as possible.

If you don't happen to be wearing a leather belt when it is time for punishment, send your sub to the closet to retrieve it. Like walking back with a switch, having your sub bring the belt to her Master and kneeling before him holding it out as an offering is the very essence of D/s.

Your belt has far more uses than simply a spanking implement. You can use it as a hand restraint, or wrap it tightly around your sub's ankles or upper thighs to hold her legs together. This simple restraint is good when you have a sub who is just beginning in bondage and wants to start with something light and familiar.

You can also wrap the belt around your sub's waist or breasts and have a "mid-body" leash to pull her around with. It is always possible for your belt to double as a makeshift leash but you want to make sure it is buckled properly so you can't pull it too tightly and accidentally restrict your sub's ability to breathe. Use the 2 fingers rule at all times when you wrap anything around your sub's neck.

## 28. Boxing Gloves

Fist mitts are gaining popularity on sites such as Sex & Submission and Kink.com. Made in metal or leather, these bulky mittens fit around the hands and lock at the wrists, leaving your sub unable to use her hands for anything. Leather fist mitts cost around $75.00 and steel globes come in at around $275. You can certainly immobilize your sub's hands and give her the feeling of total dependency for a lot less.

One of the best alternatives is boxing gloves. Traditional boxing gloves (with the mitt-like receptacle, not the MMA gloves that leave the fingers free to move) are designed to be put on by a trainer or helper. Once you get both of her hands in them and tie them tight, she really isn't able to do or hold anything with her hands.

To decrease her ability further, you can always use the tabs on the back of the gloves and connect them to each other with a lock. That way her hands are immobile and attached at the wrist. Visit any sporting goods store and you'll find boxing gloves in small sizes with a myriad of colors to choose from as well.

If you're in a hurry or purchasing boxing gloves is not within your budget (they can cost anywhere from $15 - $30 dollars), you can get a similar effect using large oven mitts. To ensure the mitts stay on you can twist cling wrap or duct tape around the base of the mitt to attach it to your sub's wrist.

If that seems bulky or awkward, have your sub make a loose fist and just use the cling wrap to wrap her hands over and over until they are nothing but plastic balls. Have scissors available in case you need to release her hands quickly.

## 29. Sleeping Bag

If immobilizing her hands is not enough and you want your sub to get the full feeling of helplessness, or simply decide to stow her for the night, a sleeping bag is a great item to pull out of the garage and into the bedroom.

Open up the sleeping bag fully and have your sub lie down on one side. Use a belt or rope to tie her calves or ankles. Restrain her hands by her side or use fist mitts of some kind to keep her from being able to unzip or manipulate the bag. Zip it up around her, leaving only her head sticking out. If it is the type with a double zipper, bring each side to her neck then tie the zippers together with string so it can't be opened or loosened without your permission.

Using a sleeping bag offers an instant immobilization tool for your sub which helps with training on permission and control. It can also be spread out beside your bed for a slave mat on those nights when you haven't granted her permission to sleep in bed with you. If you are a Daddy Dom you can buy a child's sleeping bag for your "Little" and accentuate the arena of age play.

## 30. Pool Noodles

When it comes to BDSM, there's almost nothing pool noodles can't do. You can get a long one; have your sub hold it behind her back and tie her hands around it, making a few loops with the belt of rope so that the noodle is attached to her body.

Not only is it a source of humiliation, but also a challenge to her when she's doing domestic service to have this large (but light enough to move around with) tube sticking up from behind her like a flag on a grocery cart.

The best use for pool noodles is for BDSM lifts and wedges. Many sex shops sell wedges – foam triangles you can place under a sub's hips so that her bottom is lifted into the best position for being taken from behind or spanked on the "sit spot".

Make your own wedge by putting 3 pool noodles together in triangular form and using duct tape or a strap to hold them together. You can saw the ends off so they are not too long or unwieldy. Sit the triangle on top of the bed and have your sub lay her body over the wedge. This assures you open access and gives you the best punishment angle possible.

## 31. Your Sofa

Stores and sites are full of specially made chairs, beds, mats, wedges, benches and furniture designed specifically for BDSM. While any of those are nice to have – none of those are "need to have."

The best piece of fetish furniture you could own is sitting right in front of your television. Your sofa (or couch, if you prefer) has everything you need to give your sub a good session, brutal lesson or just a nice evening to serve your needs.

For standing punishments, such as strapping, gym paddle swats, or public display, your sub can stand behind the sofa and lean over the back, exposing herself and holding on to the other side or leverage as she counts her swats or the lashes rain down on her.

To position her for rear-entry sex or more intimate spanking such as with a hairbrush, cane, small paddle or hand, require your sub to lean over the arm of the sofa. If it is too low or your sub has very long legs, use a wedge or stack of pillows to lift her bottom to the right position.

If your sofa has a recliner-like foot rest that comes up your sub can sit or kneel between the pad and the sofa, which positions her head right in front of your crotch. You can watch the game or play online effortlessly while she services you in a way befitting a sub. You can also have her lay over your lap while you read, watch or play, with her red bottom on display, ready to be spanked playfully whenever the urge arises.

# Conclusion

Overall, the most important thing to remember about BDSM is that the power is found in the relationship between a Dom and his sub. Dominance is not found in the stuff that you use, but the way you use it to train, delight, challenge, and discipline your submissive. The more creative, attentive and active you are with your sub, the more she will follow your leadership and understand your devotion is based on trust, love, and enjoyment. Look around, be inventive and most importantly – **have fun**.

**Other books by Elizabeth Cramer:**

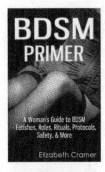

BDSM Primer - A Woman's Guide to BDSM - Fetishes, Roles, Rituals, Protocols, Safety, & More

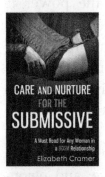

Care and Nurture for the Submissive - A Must Read for Any Woman in a BDSM Relationship

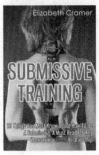

Submissive Training: 23 Things You Must Know About How To Be A Submissive. A Must Read For Any Woman In A BDSM Relationship

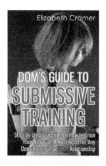
Dom's Guide To Submissive Training: Step-by-step Blueprint On How To Train Your New Sub. A Must Read For Any Dom/Master In A BDSM Relationship

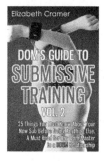
Dom's Guide To Submissive Training Vol. 2: 25 Things You Must Know About Your New Sub Before Doing Anything Else. A Must Read For Any Dom/Master In A BDSM Relationship

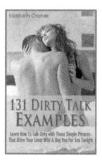
131 Dirty Talk Examples: Learn How To Talk Dirty with These Simple Phrases That Drive Your Lover Wild & Beg You For Sex Tonight

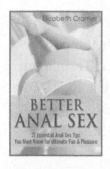
Better Anal Sex - 27 Essential Anal Sex Tips You Must Know for Ultimate Fun & Pleasure

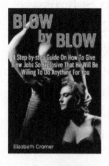
Blow By Blow - A Step-by-step Guide On How To Give Blow Jobs So Explosive That He Will Be Willing To Do Anything For You

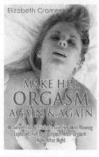
Make Her Orgasm Again and Again: 48 Simple Tips & Tricks to Give Her Mind-Blowing, Explosive, Full-Body Orgasm After Orgasm, Night After Night

Made in the USA
Las Vegas, NV
20 March 2024

87445550R00046